45 Days to Better Health

Healthy Menu Plan

Paula C. Henderson

Contents

1 Introduction

Creating a healthy diet is twofold.

One part is what you **exclude** from your diet.

The other, equally important, is what you **include** in your diet.

Who is this diet for?

This diet is for anyone who aims to be as healthy as they can for the best quality of life at any age. You do not have to have been diagnosed with any health issue to want to improve your health.

People will complain that while they followed a diet for four weeks or three months they did great, but as soon as they stopped following the diet they gained their weight back or began having health issues again.

The reason those types of diets don't work is because you stopped following them. This is why you must find a diet you can continue to follow throughout your life.

A FOREVER DIET

YOUR FOREVER DIET

The point of an elimination diet, such as this one, is to find out what your forever diet should and can look like for you.

… One of the many positive side effects for me, when I restricted gluten from my diet, was that my gray hair returned to my younger natural color of black. The dark spots, or age spots on my face and hands also disappeared. I have noticed if I cheat too often with the gluten foods I start getting the random gray hair. I get back on my strict diet and they stop coming in. It's amazing some of the unexpected benefits from this diet.

The very best outcome I did not foresee was after I went three full months without coffee (caffeine or decaf) because it's the acid, carbonated beverages, or any alcohol. See, for more than 15 years I had struggled with debilitating chronic fatigue stemming from either my hypothyroidism or my Rheumatoid Arthritis or both. But, after those three months, my fatigue was completely gone. I took up coffee again on a more limited basis, no more than 2 small cups (not mugs) restricting it to before 10 am. That was five years ago and the fatigue has never returned.

For this book I want you to just focus on being successful at following this diet for **45 consecutive days**. Hopefully, you will feel so much better it will motivate you to continue it long thereafter. Perhaps a lifetime. You will find your tolerance levels and how often you can have a cheat meal or not. This will be unique to each person.

If you go a week and a half strictly following the diet and then cheat, simply begin your 45-day count over. Day 1, Day 2, etcetera. This only works if you follow the diet for 45 days **consecutive**. It is after that you will find out your tolerance level, if any, to be able to add back any of the foods permanently or in what moderation.

Some people call this an elimination diet. Which is a fair characterization. You will eliminate certain foods for 45 consecutive days. By doing so, you will find out which foods were causing painful inflammation, headaches, stomach issues, hormonal issues, and a host of other health issues unique to you, perhaps even age spots and gray hair.

Most people are not successful on the first try or even the first few tries to go 45 consecutive days so don't beat yourself up if it takes several attempts starting over.

My own experience was quite exciting. I realized all those grains like wheat flour, corn, rice, and oats were causing my chronic constipation. It wasn't always like that. In my twenties and thirties, they helped me to be "regular". But, after I developed hypothyroidism and Rheumatoid Arthritis they affected my body differently. The doctors kept telling me to eat oatmeal and for ten years I lived on a steady diet of laxatives. Not pleasant! I had read about avoiding grains but found it hard to believe and finally realized it wouldn't hurt to try it. Bingo! Success! That was now ten years ago and I continue to avoid grains and gluten.

The most important thing to remember is that each body is different and unique in how it responds to foods. That is why these first 45 days are so very important. It may seem difficult at first but as you start to feel better and better the diet gets easier and easier. Feeling good is a great motivator.

Before you begin your "45 Days To Better Health"....

Keep in mind this diet is a process, a journey to your best health. You will find out how certain foods affect your body and your day-to-day health, if at all. If you are under a doctor's care and have diet protocols you must follow please do not vary from that.

You cannot cheat during the 45 consecutive days.
None. If you do, start over.

Do not eat anything you are allergic to. Skip those foods and instead choose a food on the diet you are not allergic to. One common complaint from people is black pepper. If you do not like black pepper or it bothers you then you should avoid it.

You should know that overeating can cause bad symptoms as much as eating bad foods. Just because it is a healthy food doesn't mean you can overeat. Having said that, if you are hungry you should eat. Just choose a small reasonable portion of healthy food.

To the point of this particular diet. You will spend 45 consecutive days only eating what is on this list. I have given you a list of foods categorized by the aisles of a standard grocery store. Then, later in the book some menu ideas as well as some recipes you can use.

The secret to this program helping you is that you stick to it for 45 consecutive days and honestly, that is the only challenging part. I know you can do it. Thousands of others have, and I have faith that you will succeed too. Remember that this is something you have chosen to do for yourself.

INSPIRED ACTION

◊ ◊ ◊ ◊ ◊ ◊

In my reading over the past year, a phrase kept coming up. Inspired Action. This resonated with me. I wrote it on a Post-it note and placed it in places I would see it throughout the day. It inspired me and it can inspire you too.

Your inspired action will depend on what you want and what you need.

Reaching for this book tells me you are looking for something. Something to help you, point you in the right direction, perhaps inspire you.

Inspired Action.

Good health; whether it be physical health or mental health should always start with a diet that works for you. Being as healthy as one can be at all ages and stages of life is essential for thriving, and succeeding, and yes, being able to tolerate the stresses and downfalls easier than an unhealthy you.

When I was in high school a classmate was involved in a horrific car accident. The doctors said she not only sustained less injury than the other victims in the car but also healed much quicker because she was in excellent physical condition at the time of the wreck. While we cannot all enjoy perfect health, I hope you will strive for your best health.

You can do this. I know you can. My motto is that there is always something to learn and always room for improvement.

Your first inspired action can be making decisions about what you eat. Deciding to move more, be more active. If you are one of the many people who feel they have difficulties in self-discipline there are some things you can do to improve.

When you make a commitment, keep it. Even and especially trivial things like if you say you are going to walk 30 minutes, walk a full 30 minutes. Don't stop at 29 minutes. If you decide you will eat lunch at 12:30 eat lunch at 12:30.

Not 12:25 or 12:45. If you say you are going to do the laundry don't stop until it is folded and put away. Don't leave it in the dryer till morning. These may seem silly and trivial but you are training your brain that you will do what you say you are going to do. The Banned Foods List is also a great exercise in self-discipline. We will get to the Banned Foods List in a later chapter. I will let you know that it is exactly what it sounds like. But, you should start now to train your brain to know that when you say you're going to do something you do it.

Much of this book is about you making decisions for yourself. I know you can make good decisions that will serve you well now and in the future. I hope you know that too.

Good eating habits:

- Choose water as your beverage with your meals.
- Chew food well.
- Do not overeat. You should try to avoid feeling overly full.
- If you are hungry you should eat something. Choose healthy.
- Avoid overly processed foods instead choose fresh whole foods.

I cannot emphasize the benefit of writing things down.

What prompted you to buy this book? Write those things down. Whether it is losing weight, having more energy, feeling less fatigue, chronic constipation, or less overall stiffness.

Now, write down ways you think might help you reach your goal. Is it eating fresh unprocessed foods? Exercising more? Not snacking? Learning to do yoga or meditations? Getting rid of that sweet tooth?

Most of us want to feel our best. We can do and want to do more things when we feel our best. We are happier and more content. If that is what you are seeking I feel certain you will find a way there. This book could be the start you needed. An inspired action. Something to do just for you that will ultimately not just benefit you but those around you.

You should feel proud of yourself. I have faith in you.

INCREASING ACTIVITY

Exercising or increasing your activity level isn't just for losing weight. It is a great stress reliever and can aid in the healing of so many other ailments. Moving is good! I encourage you to stay as active as possible or create more opportunities to be active every day.

Stand more. Stand when you fill your weekly pill box. Stand when you fold the laundry. Stand when you are making out the grocery list, or creating weekly menus. Designated exercise is the best thing you can do. At least 30 minutes six days a week. It's good for the waistline, for your heart and it's good for mental health and will help you get through stressful situations. Perhaps you can join a Pilates or yoga class, or buy a treadmill, rowing machine, elliptical, or weight bench. Start hiking in the great outdoors. You can "hike" in the city in the woods or at a park. Do more activities that involve standing and moving. Dancing is a great all-body exercise and it's fun. Walk your dog! Park further away. Start going to the grocery store again and stop with the delivery service. Get a badminton set for the yard or a basketball hoop. Go bowling.

All of these things, together with a healthier diet, make for a healthy lifestyle that will serve you well in the years to come. Studies show that people who lead healthy lifestyles are happier and deal with stressful situations better than those who do not.

I mentioned earlier that I have a treadmill. I've noticed so many people face them at the wall. I have mine faced toward my television set, you could use an iPad or tablet of course. I have at least one show that I only watch while on the treadmill. An episode is about 45 minutes long and I walk for the duration of the program. I try to choose a program that is engaging and the time flies and is over before I know it.

Just a word for those of you who want to start walking or stretching every day but can't seem to last the recommended 30 minutes.

START WHERE YOU ARE.

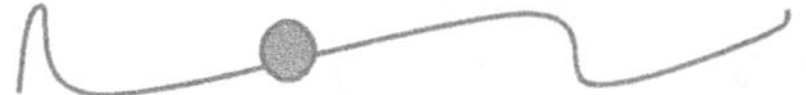

When I first started walking on my treadmill I could only walk about five minutes. But, within a week I had doubled my time and was easily walking ten and then twenty and very quickly made my way to 30 minutes. So just start. Do what you can do and build from there. I have had more than a few times in my life where I wasn't able to perform my daily exercise, due to surgery or tending to a loved one. I just started over. I had learned that with daily repetition I could very quickly get back to easily exercising a full 30 to 60 minutes each day. You will have this mastered in no time. I just know it.

Do you struggle with back pain? Back exercises, when done at least 5-6 days a week really do help! Do an internet search for back exercises. Most people find they benefit from back exercises when they are done first thing in the morning. As with any exercise routine, success depends on a consistent, repetitive exercise routine. Instead of looking at this as a chore try looking at it as time for yourself.

SUPPLEMENTS

Check all of your supplements and vitamins. Be sure none of them include soy or soybean oil. If they do, search for a brand that does not include those ingredients.

The last few chapters are suggestions for breakfast, lunch, and supper that you can choose from during your *45 Days To Better Health*. Some are simply menu ideas and there are some recipes included. Of course, don't forget about the lists above. You can choose any food from there.

But first, you will find chapters named by the aisle of your standard grocery store and a list of approved foods for each of those aisles or grocery departments. You can choose to use any of the foods listed.

BAKING AISLE

Something to remember is that gluten-free and grain-free are not the same thing. All foods that are Grain Free are gluten-free because all glutinous foods are grains, but, not all grains are glutinous.

During these 45 days you will be avoiding all grains which includes gluten but for the scant amount in some ingredients lists. If you know you are allergic to gluten and you are quite sensitive to gluten you will want to avoid products with even a scant amount.

Glutens are any foods derived from wheat. That means you should avoid these foods:

- whole wheat flour
- bleached flour
- barley
- rye
- spelt
- graham flour

Grains to avoid:

- Wheat (a gluten)
- Corn
- Rice
- Oats
- Barley
- Grits
- Cornmeal
- Popcorn
- Corn chips
- Rice flour

Foods you can have from the Baking Aisle

1. Active Dry Yeast
2. Almond Flour
3. Arrowroot (can be used in place of flour or cornstarch)
4. Baking Powder
5. Baking Soda
6. Ball Real Fruit Instant Pectin
7. Banza Pizza crusts
   Ingredients: chickpeas, water, tapioca, cocoa butter, olive oil, yeast, oregano, garlic powder, salt, date powder, sunflower lecithin, xanthan gum, baking powder
8. Bean flours
9. Bob's Red Mill Grain Free Flatbread Mix
   Ingredients: Blanched Almond flour, cassava flour, arrowroot starch, organic coconut flour, tapioca flour, salt, cream of tartar, and baking soda.
10. Buckwheat flour (made from a seed, not a grain)
11. Cacao Power
12. Cassava flour
13. Certa Pectin
14. Chebe Pizza Crust Mix
    Ingredients: Tapioca flour, modified Manioc (tapioca) flour, Iodine free salt, garlic, onion, oregano
15. Chia seeds
16. Chickpea flour
17. Cocoa powder (limit use of cocoa powder)
18. Coconut flakes
19. Coconut flour
20. Cornstarch (limit your use of cornstarch. This will replace flour for making a roux or lightly breading vegetables, meats, and seafood.
21. Extracts
22. Fava bean flour
23. Flavoring: i.e.: Vanilla, Almond, Orange, etc

24. Flax seed
25. Food coloring
26. Gelatin
27. Judee's Pea Protein Powder
28. Lentil Flour
29. Livlo Bread Loaf: keto baking mix
     Ingredients: almonds, tapioca fiber, ground flaxseed,
     baking powder, sea salt

30. Natures Charm Evaporated Coconut Milk (canned)
31. Nut flours
32. Nuts
33. Pork Panko
34. Psyllium husk
35. Salt
36. Seeds
37. Shredded coconut
38. Tapioca starch
39. Tiger Nut flour
40. Wilton Clear Imitation Butter Flavoring
41. Wine sherry
42. Xanthan gum

Oil and NonStick Cooking Spray

Use oils sparingly. No deep-fried foods. Use oils to toss a salad, brush onto bread in place of butter, toss/drizzle vegetables that you will bake. If your baked chicken is dry it's because you overcooked it. Baked chicken should be moist and juicy and you do not have to baste it.

Avoid oils that say "Vegetable Oil". If you will look at the ingredients list it is soybean oil.

1. Almond Oil
2. Avocado Oil
3. Black Truffle Oil
4. Canola oil
5. Coconut oil
6. Grapeseed oil
7. Hemp Seed Oil
8. Nut oils
9. Olive oil
10. Palm Oil
11. Peanut Oil
12. Safflower oil
13. Sesame oil
14. Sunflower oil
15. Walnut oil

SEASONING AND SPICE

During the first 45 days, you will be avoiding nightshades for the most part. If you already know you are sensitive to nightshades, even scant amounts in an ingredient list then you should continue to avoid them altogether.

Nightshades to avoid include:

- White and red potatoes. (All potatoes except sweet potatoes)
- Eggplant
- Tomatoes and tomato products
- Bell peppers
- Hot Peppers and by-products like hot sauce
- Nightshade spices like crushed red pepper and paprika

Stay away from anything with paprika chili powder or peppers. Stay away from those blends that say spicy. Do not rely on the front verbiage. Be sure to get into the habit of reading the actual ingredients list on the back. Reading the label is very important. The brand Dash has a few blends listed here, but their Lemon-Pepper has cayenne pepper. There are a few Lemon-Pepper blends listed that are 'clean'.

If you tend to use a lot of paprika, a nightshade, try using cumin instead. If you smell the cumin, you will find it smells much like paprika!

1. Allspice
2. Anise
3. Aroma One Organics Basil Puree (tube, like paste)
4. Aroma One Organics Ginger Puree (tube, like paste)
5. Basil
6. Bay Leaf
7. Bragg Nutritional Yeast
8. Celery Salt
9. Celery Seed

10. Cinnamon
11. Coriander
12. Cumin
13. Dash Everything But the Salt Seasoning Blend
    Ingredients: dried garlic, dried onion, sesame seeds, poppy seeds.

14. Dash Salt-Free Garlic & Herb Seasoning Blend
    Ingredients: dried garlic, dried onion, sesame seeds, poppy seeds.

15. Dill weed
16. Dried Mushroom Powder (packet)
17. Extracts and flavorings
18. Fennel
19. Frontier Co-Op Five Spice Powder – Awaken
    Ingredients: cinnamon, fennel, cloves, star anise, white pepper

20. Frontier Co-Op Garam Marsala Seasoning
    Ingredients: cardamom, cinnamon, cloves, cumin, black pepper, coriander

21. Frontier Co-op Herbes De Provence
    Ingredients: savory, thyme, rosemary, basil, tarragon, lavender flowers

22. Frontier Co-Op Za'atar Seasoning
    Ingredients: hyssop, sesame seeds, sumac berries and salt, thyme, sea salt.

    [Hyssop is an edible member of the mint family and is safe to eat. Lore tells us that hyssop used to be used as a natural medicinal remedy for conditions like asthma, sore throat, stomach upset, and infections.]

23. Garlic powder
24. Garlic salt
25. Great Value Everything Bagel Seasoning
    Ingredients: sesame seeds, salt, dehydrated garlic, dehydrated onion, black sesame seeds, poppy seeds

26. Great Value Italian Seasoning
      Ingredients: basil, oregano, rosemary, thyme, parsley, garlic

27. Ground ginger
28. Kinder's Seasoning The Blend
      Ingredients: sea salt, dehydrated garlic, black pepper, sunflower oil, garlic oil

29. Lemon Peel
30. Lemon Zest
31. Mace
32. Marjoram
33. McCormick You Crack Me Up Egg Topping Seasoning
      Ingredients: salt, black pepper, garlic, onion and celery seed

34. McCormick Lemon & Pepper Seasoning
      Ingredients: salt, black pepper, citric acid, onion, sugar, garlic, calcium stearate, silicon dioxide and calcium silicate, celery seed, lemon oil, and FD&C Yellow No 5 Lake.

      *This product does have a few artificial ingredients for those of you who are avoiding those 100%

35. McCormick Organic Poultry Seasoning
      Ingredients: organic thyme, organic sage, organic marjoram, organic rosemary, organic black pepper, and organic nutmeg.

36. Minced Garlic in water
37. Minced onion
38. Morton Natures Seasons Seasoning Blend. (Be aware one of the ingredients says spices. This could be anything. Since this is a food product used sparingly I would say give it a try, but, be mindful if it causes you problems. Spices can oftentimes mean paprika, which is a nightshade.)
39. Nutmeg

40. Onion powder
41. Oregano
42. Reese Anchovy Past (tube)
> Ingredients: wild-caught anchovies, olive oil, salt.
43. Rosemary
44. Rum extract
45. Sage
46. Salt
47. Solo Pure Almond Paste (box)
48. Thyme
49. Turmeric
50. Vanilla Bean

BEVERAGES

During your 45 Days to Better Health, you may choose any of the following beverages:

1.   Water: Water should be the beverage you drink the majority of the time. I was having lots of stomach issues and after trying many different types of water and water filters I found Distilled Water did not bother me.

     Begin making it a habit to always choose water with your meals.

2.   Dairy-free milk that does not contain sugar, soy, or oats.

*   Cashew milk
*   Coconut milk
*   Decaffeinated herbal teas are okay so long as you do not sweeten them. Teas like green tea, Chamomile, and ginger are okay.
*   Unsweetened Almond Milk
*   Unsweetened Vanilla Almond Milk

3.   Carrot Juice without any sweetener.
4.   Celery Juice, again nothing added.
5.   Cucumber Water

Most people find they take to the dairy-free milk just fine. I did not, but, I never like regular dairy milk either. I can tell you that I acquired a taste for it very quickly so if you, like me, do not favor unsweetened almond milk don't give up. I started by just sipping a tiny bit a few times a day. Within one week I was able to easily drink an entire glass and found I enjoyed it very much. My favorite, regardless of brand, is the unsweetened vanilla almond milk.

During the 45 days please avoid regular and decaf coffee, not just because of the caffeine as much as because of the acid. This means not even decaffeinated coffee. I am a big coffee drinker so for me this was a real challenge. I can tell you it was worth it and I still occasionally restrict my coffee for a month or so at a time. Last year I was experiencing some stomach issues and decided to restrict my coffee, carbonated beverages, and alcohol for a month. This turned into three full months without any coffee, soda, or alcohol. After the first month, I could tell it was helping and felt if I continued another month it would be very beneficial. It turned into three months at which I realized not only was my stomach issues gone but the chronic fatigue I had experienced for over ten years was completely gone. After those three months, I did go back to drinking coffee but not carbonated beverages or alcohol. I added those to my **Banned Foods list**. I also no longer drink coffee on an empty stomach. This may help you as well.

Avoid any sweeteners including natural or artificial during your 45 days.

Avoid all juices.

You can have very healthy bone broth.

BREAD, CRACKERS, TACO SHELLS

You will be avoiding gluten during these 45 days. Foods like bread, pasta, and dry cereal. Gluten can also be symptomatic to many people, causing hives, headaches, brain fog, triggering those who struggle with depression or sadness, and inflammation in the gut and/or joints.

You will also be avoiding grains like corn, oats, and rice. All are high-carb foods.

These grain-free options are still high-carb foods and highly processed. You will want to track when you consume one of these foods and limit your consumption to just two servings a week.

Here are some grain-free gluten-free foods to choose from:

1. Against the Grain Pita Bread

    Ingredients: Tapioca Starch, Water, Buckwheat flour, olive oil, milk, salt, raisin juice concentrate, yeast.

    *This has milk. Since it is the fifth ingredient of just eight total ingredients that tells us it is one of the least of the ingredients. If you cannot have any dairy you will want to avoid this food.

2. Simple Mills Bread Mix

    Ingredients: Almond flour, arrowroot, flax meal, tapioca, sea salt, baking soda

3. Against The Grain Cinnamon Raisin Bagels

    Ingredients: Tapioca starch, organic coconut milk, eggs, canola oil, raisins, salt, cinnamon.

4. Siete Almond Flour Grain-Free Tortillas

    Ingredients: almond flour, tapioca flour, water, sea salt, xanthan gum

5. Siete Taco Shells

    Ingredients: cassava flour and cassava starch, avocado oil, pumpkin seed meal, pumpkin powder, psyllium husk powder, sea salt.

6. Simple Mills Muffin Mixes

Avoid the Chocolate flavor, but you can enjoy the Vanilla, Pumpkin, and Banana. There are other Grain Free muffin mixes out there but they always have complaints of being too sweet tasting and I agree.

BUTTER

There is no getting around the fact that dairy-free butter is highly processed. Limit the use of these products as much as possible.

Oh, the butter. Dairy-free butter is a highly processed food but we include it as it is used sparingly. You can use real butter and make ghee or you can purchase ghee in a jar at some markets or online. Here, I will list the dairy-free butter you can find in grocery stores.

You will notice I have the lecithin highlighted because I know some people avoid those, we use butter minimally and most people find they can tolerate it just fine. This is something you will have to decide for yourself and your own needs.

'I Can't Believe It's Not Butter with Olive Oil' includes soybean oil. So this product is not approved for this list.

1. Country Crock Dairy Free Avocado Oil Plant Butter Sticks
   Ingredients: blend of palm fruit, palm kernel, canola and avocado oil, water salt, pea protein, sunflower **lecithin**, citric acid, vitamin A palmitate, natural flavor, beta carotene ****Contains lecithin and the label says may contain soy.*

2. Earth Balance Soy Free Spread
   Ingredients: oil blend of palm fruit, canola, safflower, flax and olive oils. Salt, natural pea protein, flavor, sunflower **lecithin**, lactic acid (non-dairy), and naturally extracted annatto

   ****Alert lecithin**

3. Miyoko's European Style Cultured Vegan Butter
   Ingredients: organic coconut oil, organic cultured cashew milk, filtered water, organic sunflower oil, organic sunflower lecithin, sea salt

***Includes lecithins**

4. Simple Truth Organic Dairy-Free Salted Butter
   Ingredients: Prepared Butter Beans (Water, Organic Butter Beans), Vegetable Oil Blend (Organic Coconut Oil and Organic Sunflower Oil), Sea Salt, Cultured Dextrose, Calcium Citrate, Natural Flavors, Sunflower Lecithin, Organic Konjac Root Powder, Mixed Tocopherols, Annatto, Caramel Color

5. Violife Plant Butter
   Ingredients: plant-based oil blend of canola, coconut, and sunflower oils, water, sunflower **lecithin**, fava bean protein, citric acid, natural flavor, glucose, beta carotene for color.

   ***Lecithin**

'Vegan' implies dairy-free as it would exclude animal byproducts. 'Grain Free' implies gluten-free as all glutens are grains.

CHEESE

During your *45 Days To Better Health,* we will all but eliminate cheese, but for scant amounts in a very limited number of food products listed. Avoid completely if you can. For those of you who cannot fathom going without cheese for 45 consecutive days, I encourage you to make a list of all the foods you like that you never eat cheese on, or that you would be fine without. For example:

- Seafood
- Chicken
- Meatloaf
- Roasted vegetables
- Baked sweet potato
- Nuts and seeds
- Berries and watermelon

You get the idea.

CONDIMENTS

During the 45 consecutive days, you will be avoiding ketchup, hot sauce ready-made salad dressings, barbecue sauce, steak sauce, taco sauce, prepared tartar sauce (you can easily make your own), or any other condiments with soybean oil, dairy, or nightshades.

- Capers
- Coconut Aminos (a healthy substitute for soy sauce)
- Horseradish that does not have soybean oil. Choose a brand like Silver Spring Prepared Horseradish. The ingredients are horseradish, vinegar, water, salt, and natural flavor.
- Kitchen Bouquet Browning Seasoning Sauce: caramel color, water, vegetable base (water, carrots, celery, cabbage, onion, parsley, turnips, parsnips), Less than 2% of spices, salt, sodium benzoate added to preserve freshness.
- Liquid Smoke: water, natural hickory smoke flavor, vinegar, molasses, caramel color, salt.
- Mayo: a brands list with ingredients is listed below within this chapter.
- Mustard: many people will avoid mustard if they are avoiding nightshades. The ingredients in most standard mustards are: Distilled vinegar, water, mustard seed, salt, turmeric, paprika, spice, natural flavor, and garlic powder. That is the ingredients list from French's Classic Yellow Mustard. Paprika and *spices are the culprits here. They are not first on the list so there is not only a scant amount in each serving but generally when a person eats mustard it is in small amounts. Most find they tolerate mustard fine but, of course, if you find it bothers you, then you should avoid it.
- Sesame Oil
- Tahini: Ingredients: roasted ground sesame seeds
- Thai Kitchen Fish Sauce: Ingredients are anchovies, salt, water, and sugar.
- Vinegar (all except Malt Vinegar)

Dips

Guacamole and Hummus. As a reminder, Hummus is made from legumes, aka Chick Peas, sometimes called Garbanzo Beans. If you are avoiding legumes stick to guacamole. Another dip would be refried beans. Just heat up in a saucepan stirring very well, and add some lime juice. Goes great with grain-free crackers, celery, and cauliflower florets. Remember that legumes are a very high-carb food so be sure to limit servings of legumes to just once or twice a week.

Mayo

- Chosen Foods Classic Mayo
  Ingredients: Avocado Oil, water, egg yolks, whole eggs, distilled white vinegar, mustard and mustard seed, salt, spices, and rosemary extract.

  *Mustard generally includes some paprika. Almost everyone can tolerate the tiny amount included in the small amount of mayo one would consume in this product. However, I know there are some who are extremely sensitive to paprika, a nightshade, and if that is you then please avoid this product.

- Hellman's Canola Oil Mayonnaise
  Ingredients: water, canola oil, food starch (corn, potato), sugar, eggs, vinegar, salt, lemon juice concentrate, sorbic acid, calcium disodium, paprika, vitamin E, beta carotene

  *potato and cornstarch

- Hellman's Plant-Based Mayo
  Ingredients: canola oil, water, modified food starch (potato and corn starch), distilled vinegar, less than 2% sugar, salt, lemon juice concentrate, sorbic acid and calcium disodium, paprika extract

  *A bit of potato and corn starch.

- Just Mayo No Egg Plant-Based
    Ingredients: Canola Oil, water, white distilled vinegar, lemon juice concentrate, modified food starch, pea protein, salt, spice sugar, fruit and vegetable juice for color, and calcium disodium – a preservative.

    *Scant amounts of food starch, spices, and sugar.

- Sir Kensington's Vegan Mayo
    Ingredients: sunflower oil, aquafaba (water and chickpeas), lemon juice, coconut sugar, salt, vinegar, acacia gum, rosemary extract, xanthan gum, black pepper, citric acid, mustard extract, and lemon oil.

- Tamarind Paste
    Ingredients: tamarind concentrate

Tamarind has a unique sweet and sour flavor. Some people say it tastes tangy and tart and others think it has a sour taste. One person described it as if she had mixed lemon, dates, and a bit of apricot.

Tamarind is often used in place of barbecue sauce. This doesn't mean it tastes just like a BBQ sauce but it is a good substitute to creating a tasty chicken.

EGGS

- Fresh eggs prepared any way
- Liquid egg whites
- Egg Beaters
- Dried Whole Egg Powder
- Pre-packaged boiled eggs

FROZEN FOODS

All the vegetables listed in the produce section of this book that are frozen are approved. If you have not perused your frozen foods section of vegetables lately you are missing a lot! Take your time one day and look at all of the sections to see if you find some new products that make cooking and meal preparation a bit more convenient. There is now frozen avocado, and frozen riced cauliflower, great for those with arthritis or time constraints! Frozen fresh sliced mushrooms and more. If you hate canned asparagus don't let that keep you from trying the frozen asparagus spears! Spread them on a sheet pan, drizzle with oil and salt, and bake until golden brown, simply boil as a side dish, or add to soups and sauces.

Frozen Fruits

- Berries
- Blackberries
- Blueberries
- Melon
- Raspberries
- Strawberries

During your 45 consecutive days please limit frozen fruits to just those on this list.

Frozen Vegetables

Avoid the frozen Edamame beans. These are soybeans. Avoid soybean and soy products during this time.

Remember that all vegetables are gluten-free, dairy-free, soy-free, and nightshade-free except:

White and red potatoes are nightshades
Sweet potatoes and yams are okay to eat.

Eggplant is a nightshade
Edamame beans are soybeans
Tomatoes and tomatillos are nightshades
All peppers, red – green – yellow are nightshades
Onions are okay to eat unless they bother your stomach

1. Asparagus
2. Birds Eye Normandy blend Vegetables
3. Birds Eye Oven Roasters Brussels Sprouts & Carrots:
   > Ingredients: Brussels sprouts, carrots, sea salt, and herbs
4. Birds Eye Shredded Veggies Carrots & Broccoli Florets
5. Birds Eye Shredded Veggies White Cabbage and Carrots
   > Ingredients: white cabbage, carrots, scallions, grilled onions, extra virgin olive oil, salt, black pepper, sunflower oil
6. Birds Eye Steamfresh Broccoli Carrots Sugar Snap Peas & Water
7. Broccoli
8. Brussels Sprouts
9. Butternut squash
10. Carrots
11. Cauliflower
12. Chestnuts
13. Collard greens
14. Frozen herbs
15. Frozen whole okra
16. Garlic
17. Green beans
18. Green Giant Riced Veggies Broccoli
19. Green Giant Riced Veggies Cauliflower
    > Ingredients: cauliflower
20. Green Giant Rainbow Cauliflower
    > Ingredients: cauliflower
21. Green Giant Riced Veggies Cauliflower & Broccoli Blend
    > Ingredients: cauliflower, broccoli, olive oil, garlic,

basil, parsley, sea salt

22. Green Giant Riced Veggies Cauliflower & Sweet Potato
23. Green Giant Riced Veggies Cauliflower, with lemon and garlic
24. Green Giant Riced Veggies: Cauliflower Medley
    Ingredients: Cauliflower, green peas, onion, carrots, green onion

25. Green Giant Riced Veggies: Cauliflower Risotto Medley
    Ingredients: cauliflower, green peas, onion, carrots, green onion

26. Green Giant Veggie Spirals: Zucchini
    Ingredients: zucchini

27. Kale
28. Mushrooms
29. Onions
30. Peas
31. Riced Cauliflower
32. Snow peas
33. Spaghetti Squash
34. Spinach
35. Sugar snap peas
36. Sweet Potatoes
37. Turnip greens
38. Zucchini Squash sliced Blend

Miscellaneous Frozen Foods

1. Banza Pizza crust
    Ingredients: chickpeas, water, tapioca, cocoa butter, olive oil, yeast, oregano, garlic powder, salt, date powder, sunflower **lecithin**, xanthan gum, baking powder,

    *****lecithin**

2. Outer Aisle Cauliflower Pizza Crust and Wraps
    Ingredients: fresh cauliflower, whole cage-free eggs, **parmesan cheese**, nutritional yeast, garlic basil, oregano.

    *This product contains **dairy**.

Just a reminder that just because a package says it is a Cauliflower Pizza Crust does not mean it is gluten-free, grain-free, and/or soy-free so be sure to check your ingredients list if you want to purchase one.

Frozen Meat

Just a reminder that you will see the word *spice or *spices as an ingredient list in prepared foods. This vague term may or may not include things like paprika, red bell pepper, and other types of nightshades you may want to avoid. You will have to decide for yourself if these individual food products cause you a problem or not. If the food product is described as spicy that would be a clue that there are some nightshades included. Other keywords to avoid are chipotle, Italian, hot, fajita, or Mexican flavored.

1. Butterball All Natural White Turkey Burger
        Ingredients: white turkey, sea salt, natural flavoring

2. Great Value 100% Pure Beef Burgers: the only ingredient is beef.
3. Hamburger Patties: unseasoned. The only ingredient should be beef.
4. HEB Original Beef Burgers
5. HEB Seasoned Turkey Burgers
6. Meijer 100% Beef Ground Beef Burgers
7. Meijer Lean Turkey Burgers
8. Sams Choice 100% Angus Beef Burgers
9. Steak-Umms: The ingredient is just beef. That's it.

FRUIT

Fruits have natural sugars so you will want to keep them at a minimum, but there are a few we can have on a limited basis so long as you can enjoy them without any sweetener.

Most fruits should be avoided but here are a few. I suggest only eating a small serving of the following fruits no more than twice a week during the first 45 days.

- Blackberries
- Blueberries
- Citrus fruits like oranges, lemons, and limes.
- Honeydew
- Raspberries
- Strawberries
- Watermelon

LEGUMES

If you have legumes, have it at a ratio of just ¼ of your vegetables or protein. Three-fourths of your plate should be true vegetables or protein and just one-fourth of legumes.

Legumes are:

- Black beans
- Garbanzo beans
- Red beans
- Northern beans
- Pinto beans
- Black Eyed Peas
- Navy Beans

MEAT

You can have meats but limit them to a small serving just every other day for one meal. Be sure they are not breaded. It is best to choose whole meats as you find in the Meat Department but there are exceptions and I have made you a list. There were a few in the previous chapter for frozen foods.

If you are a vegetarian and looking for meat-free substitutes like Impossible, Beyond brand, and other plant-based meat substitutes, be mindful that many of them use soy protein which you will want to avoid. Some of them also use nightshades to season some of the foods and food starches that you may be avoiding.

The Beyond Meat brand uses wheat and it will state on the packaging that it contains wheat. Gardein Plant Based Beef Crumbles uses soy protein so you will also want to avoid that. As far as I can tell all of the Morning Star products use not only wheat flour but also soy. The Ultimate Plant Based Burger Patties also use wheat; a gluten.

Tofu is a soybean product. To be avoided.

Here is a list of approved meats.

1. Beef: ground beef or steak
2. Beef roast
3. Brisket
4. Chicken: ground chicken, pieces, whole. With or without bone
5. Chicken gizzards
6. Chicken skin
7. Corned beef
8. Duck
9. Fowl
10. Game meat
11. Gizzards
12. Ground beef
13. Ground chicken
14. Ground pork
15. Ground turkey
16. Hen

17. Lamb
18. Liver
19. Neck bones
20. Oxtail
21. Pigs Feet
22. Pork: ground, chops, roast
23. Pork Chitterlings
24. Pork chop
25. Pork roast
26. Pork steaks
27. Ribs
28. Steak
29. Stew meat

You will be avoiding lunchmeats during your 45 days. A very limited amount of uncured meats would be okay in very small servings but avoid all altogether or keep it at a bare minimum.

PACKAGED SALADS

Lots of pre-made salads these days. Skip that dressing, the fake bacon bits and choose those bags without cheese or tomatoes.

Some examples that are okay to eat:

- Butter Lettuce Salad
- Broccoli slaw
- Classic Iceberg Salad
- Romaine salad
- Shredded Coleslaw – no dressing just shredded cabbage and carrots
- Spinach
- Spring mix

Any green salad mix with just approved, 'clean' vegetables included.

- Taylor Farms, Dole, Mann's, Little Leaf Farms, and Marketside are just a few of the companies that make several chopped salad kits in a bag. You will find these in the produce department.
- Marketside Super Blend in a bag includes Brussels sprouts, Napa cabbage, kohlrabi, broccoli, carrots, and kale.

Beware the Caesar Salad bags as they have croutons and parmesan cheese as well as usually a dressing you should avoid.

I have noticed more and more dressings inside these salad kits are using sunflower or canola oil. Be careful though, some still use soybean oil.

PASTA

If you have pasta, have it at a ratio of just ¼ of your vegetables or protein. Three-fourths of your plate should be vegetables or protein and just one-fourth pasta.

1. Banza Brand Pasta
        Ingredients: chickpeas, tapioca, pea protein, xanthan gum. (this is my favorite brand of pasta and it is at all my local grocery stores.)

2. Jovial Grain Free Cassava Fusilli
        Ingredients: cassava flour, water

3. Palmini Hearts of Palm Lasagna noodles (pouch or can)
        Ingredients: sliced hearts of palm, water, sea salt, citric acid.

SAUCES

1. Primal Kitchen No Dairy Alfredo Sauce (jar)
    Ingredients: water, avocado oil, tapioca starch, organic pumpkin seed butter, roasted garlic, sea salt, onion powder, lemon juice concentrate, black pepper, citric acid, nutritional yeast, and a negligible amount of sugar.

2. Seggiano Fresh Basil Pesto (*this brand does not have parmesan cheese*)
    Ingredients: olive oil, cashew nuts, fresh basil, sea salt, pine nuts.

3. La Dee Da Gourmet Cauliflower Alfredo Style Sauce
    Ingredients: water, cauliflower, cauliflower powder, nutritional yeast, garlic powder, sea salt, xanthan gum, black pepper, and lactic acid.

4. La Dee Da Savory Mushroom Basil Sauce
    Ingredients: water, cremini mushroom, button mushroom, onions, extra virgin olive oil, sweet potato, chickpea flour, garlic, basil, sea salt, xanthan gum, black pepper, sage, lactic acid.

5. Primal Kitchen No-Dairy White Pizza Sauce
    Ingredients: water, pumpkin seed butter, avocado oil, organic roasted garlic, tapioca starch, sea salt, onion powder, lemon juice concentrate, citric acid, nutritional yeast, black pepper, dried oregano, dried basil, dried marjoram, crushed red pepper.

    *Crushed red pepper is a nightshade. I included this product because this ingredient is listed last meaning there is a negligible amount. If you already know that you are very sensitive to any nightshades or red peppers please avoid this product.

SEAFOOD

Seafood is very healthy and you can have seafood as often as you want. The only criteria is to avoid breaded fish and sushi. Do not consume raw fish during this time. You can pick it back up after the 45 days. Also, lots of the sushi dishes contain rice, a grain, and/or soy sauce which we are also avoiding during your 45 Days To Better Health.

Fresh Seafood

1. Ahi
2. Calamari (no breading)
3. Catfish
4. Cod
5. Crab Legs
6. Crawfish
7. Halibut
8. Lobster
9. Mackerel
10. Mussels
11. Ocean Perch
12. Oysters
13. Perch
14. Scallops
15. Shark
16. Shrimp
17. Smelt
18. Snapper
19. Swai
20. Swordfish
21. Tilapia
22. Trout
23. Tuna fillet
24. Whiting

Canned Seafood

1. Bumble Bee Skinless Boneless Smoked Trout
       Ingredients: smoked trout fillets, canola oil, salt.

2. Chicken of the Sea Chub Mackerel in Brine
       Ingredients: mackerel, water, salt

3. Chicken of the Sea Whole Oysters
       Ingredients: whole oysters, water, salt.

4. Cod Liver
5. Deming's Red Sockeye Salmon
       Ingredients: red sockeye salmon and salt

6. Great Value Alaskan Pink Salmon
       Ingredients: salmon, water, salt

7. Great Value Chunk Light Tuna in Water
       Ingredients: light tuna, water, vegetable broth

8. Great Value Smoked Oysters
       Ingredients: oysters, cottonseed oil, salt

9. King Oscar Skinless & Boneless Mackerel Fillets in Olive Oil
       Ingredients: skinless and boneless North Atlantic
       mackerel, olive oil, salt.

10. Pampa Mackerel in brine
       Ingredients: mackerel, water, salt.

11. Polar Kipper Snacks
       Ingredients: all natural smoked boneless fillets of
       Herring, water, and salt.

12. Reese Large Smoked Oysters
       Ingredients: smoked oysters, cottonseed oil, salt.

13. Safe Catch Wild Albacore Tuna
       Ingredients: albacore tuna, salt.

14. Season Mackerels Skinless and Boneless in Olive Oil
       Ingredients: mackerel, olive oil, salt.

15. Starkist Chunk Light Tuna in Water
       Ingredients: light tuna, water, vegetable broth, salt.

16. Starkist skinless boneless pink salmon
       Ingredients: pink salmon, water, salt

SNACKS

See Bread and Crackers for CRACKERS.

1. Chicharrones
   Ingredients: fried pork rinds, salt added

2. Fried Pork Skins
3. Siete Grain Free Tortilla Chips
   Ingredients: cassava flour, avocado oil, pumpkin powder, coconut flour, psyllium husk powder, sea salt

4. Simple Mills Almond Flour Crackers – Sea Salt
   Ingredients: Nut and seed flour blend of almonds, sunflower seeds, and flax seeds. Tapioca starch, cassava flour, sunflower oil, sea salt, onion, garlic, rosemary extract,

5. Simple Mills Soft Baked Almond Flour Bars Dark Chocolate
   This product has a small amount of cane sugar and molasses but they do not have a heavy sweet taste. This is one reason I like this brand over some of the others. Please eat sparingly, not every day, if at all.

   Ingredients: Almond flour, coconut four, coconut nectar, sunflower flour, flax flour, chia flour, chocolate chips (cane sugar, unsweetened chocolate cocoa butter), tapioca starch, coconut oil, almond butter, molasses, egg whites, raisin juice, sea salt, baking soda, rosemary extract.

MISCELLANEOUS FOODS

MUSHROOMS: Fresh mushrooms are best and there are many varieties with their very own taste and texture. But frozen mushrooms are also okay, just be sure to choose unbreaded, plain frozen mushrooms.

Fresh mushrooms: White mushrooms, baby Bella, whole brown mushrooms, Portabella mushroom caps, Cremini mushrooms

1. Green Giant Mushrooms (Jar)

    Ingredients: mushrooms, water, salt, ascorbic acid to maintain color.

    I did not list any other brands, jars, or cans, because this was the only one I found that did not include Citric Acid. Limiting your citric acid is encouraged during this time.

Olives

All olives are okay. Remove the pimento if it is a pimento-stuffed green olive.

- Black olives
- Kalamata olives
- Green olives

Broth

To use as a base for soups, gravy, and sauces.

A caution to not assume all broth is just broth. Check your labels.

NUTS AND SEEDS

I like nuts and seeds in a bowl with Almond milk. I eat it with a spoon like I would cereal.

1. Almonds
2. Brazil
3. Cashews
4. Chestnuts
5. Chia Seeds
6. Coconut
7. Flax Seeds
8. Hazelnuts
9. Macadamia
10. Peanuts (*peanuts are a pulse aka legume)
11. Pecans
12. Pepitas
13. Pine Nuts
14. Pistachios
15. Poppy seeds
16. Pumpkin seeds
17. Sesame seeds
18. Sunflower seeds
19. Walnuts

VEGETABLES

Fresh vegetables from the produce department are the very best choice. I feel my best when I focus on these foods over any other. Having said that frozen is acceptable and canned is okay but keep the canned at a minimum. Try to incorporate foods from the produce department as often as you can. Preferably as a part of your daily diet.

The Produce Department is Your Best Friend

Did You Know?

Some would go so far as to say that dark leafy greens are the most healthy food one can consume. Many refer to leafy greens as a superfood. Incorporating green leafy foods under, on top, and beside as many meals as possible is a great thing to do for your body.

Green leafy vegetables are a great source of vitamins C, E, K, iron, calcium, potassium, and magnesium. They also offer the body beta carotene, which the body breaks down into Vitamin A. Cooked or raw, you can't go wrong with leafy greens on your plate.

I have created a list of vegetables you can consume during your 45 consecutive days.

Packaged Salads are above in their own category.

1. Acorn squash
2. All leafy greens
3. Artichokes
4. Arugula
5. Asparagus
6. Avocados (technically a fruit but…)
7. Basil
8. Bok Choy
9. Broccoli
10. Broccoli Raab

11. Broccolini
12. Brussels sprouts
13. Butter Lettuce
14. Butternut squash
15. Cabbage
16. Carrots
17. Cauliflower
18. Celery
19. Chard
20. Chayote Squash
21. Chicory
22. Chinese Cabbage
23. Chives
24. Cilantro
25. Collard Greens
26. Cress
27. Cucumbers
28. Daikon
29. Endive
30. Fennel
31. Fiddleheads
32. Frisee
33. Garlic
34. Ginger root
35. Green beans
36. Green onions
37. Green peas
38. Herbs
39. Horseradish root
40. Iceberg lettuce
41. Jicama
42. Kale
43. Kraut
44. Kohlrabi
45. Leeks
46. Lettuce
47. Mushrooms
48. Mustard Greens
49. Nettles

50. Okra
51. Onions
52. Oregano
53. Parsley
54. Parsnips
55. Peas
56. Pumpkin
57. Purple Cabbage
58. Radicchio
59. Radishes
60. Rhubarb
61. Romaine lettuce
62. Rosemary
63. Rutabaga
64. Savoy Cabbage
65. Scallions
66. Shallots
67. Snow peas
68. Spaghetti squash
69. Spinach
70. Squash
71. Sugar Snap peas
72. Sweet potato

VINEGAR

1. Alessi Raspberry Blush White Vinegar
2. Apple Cider Vinegar
3. Balsamic Vinegar
4. Distilled White Vinegar
5. Organic Coconut Vinegar
6. Pickling vinegar
7. Red wine vinegar
8. Vinegar: (all vinegar except Malt Vinegar. Malt vinegar is a gluten)
9. White wine vinegar

YOGURT

Yogurt can be very healthy, even dairy-free yogurts. During your 45 Days to Better Health stick to plain yogurt. You can eat it alone, or eat it with berries or nuts. Just resist any urge to add sweetener.

- Forager Project Cashewmilk Yogurt
- Silk Almondmilk dairy-free yogurt
- So Delicious Dairy Free Coconutmilk Yogurt alternative

Not all dairy-free yogurt is okay. Many have soybean oil, or soy protein in the ingredients list. You will want to avoid that. If your grocery store has a plain yogurt brand not mentioned here that is dairy-free and soy-free you should consider that okay to consume.

This list will not include dairy-free ice creams as there are no benefits to outweigh the sugar content in that particular food. Avoid dairy-free ice creams and frozen treats during this time.

45-Day Menu Ideas

In the next few chapters, you will see food choices and recipes for breakfast, lunch, and supper. Each day choose one from each group for each meal or come up with your own from the lists in the previous chapters. There is also a chapter for condiments recipes that are used in some of the breakfasts, lunch, and supper meals.

My suggestion is to just keep it simple these next 6 weeks. Eggs, nuts, and berries for breakfast. Or, choose from the approved muffin and bagel choices once or twice a week.

Supper leftovers for lunch or a salad. Even your evening meal can be quick, easy, and delicious. Go for some sautéed vegetables and baked fish or chicken or a stir-fry. There are lots of choices in the previous chapters and the ones that follow. Read through them carefully and create your own menu ideas lists while you do. I am including some recipes if you want to try them but the best way to embrace a restricted diet is to keep it as simple as possible.

Let's also start a Banned Foods List.

Starting to make healthier choices can be as simple as choosing water for all your meals from now on and saying no to dessert and dinner rolls.

Banned Foods List

Banned Foods List. It sounds daunting but I have found throughout the years of being a weight loss counselor and nutritionist that people like it and find it works well for them. I hope you will find that too.

The Banned Foods List started years ago after reading an article in a magazine. Julia Louis Dreyfus was being interviewed as she had just turned 40 years old. She shared that she had recently gone to the doctor for an annual checkup. Her takeaway from the doctor's advice that day stayed with her. The doctor told her it wasn't too late to get as healthy as she could be, to be as healthy as one could be, and that she should always strive for that. This resonated with her because she had just never given it much thought like many of us in our twenties and thirties who take our resilient health for granted. Everything in moderation though, right? No. Actually no.

In moderation keeps so many people in an unhealthy state and has sabotaged so many otherwise well-meaning efforts to improve one's health. My personal story with the "in moderation" mantra was that in my mid to late thirties I began my healthier lifestyle journey for perhaps the third or fourth time. My teenage daughter had started a part-time job at the video store and worked primarily evening. As she wasn't home for supper I could do whatever I wanted. Yeah! It was going well, I was feeling better, and looking better. I had even lost about 15 pounds. But, I wasn't where I wanted to be or thought I could be. It was also during this time I purchased my first treadmill and I have had a treadmill ever since. I was, at the time, exercising my "in moderation" rights and while I ate very healthy throughout the week I did allow myself freedom over the weekends and the occasional pastry donuts that invariably showed up at work on Fridays.

After several months of being stuck, I decided to ban the donuts and pastry at work. I would just say no. These foods had no place in my diet. I haven't eaten one since. That was over 20 years ago. Although I recall how wonderful they tasted I can tell you honestly that I do not miss them. I lost another five pounds or so and I felt much better. I was less fatigued and less bloated. I had banned them for life and I stuck to it. I can't tell you how good I felt about this. I knew all that overly processed sugar and flour was not healthy for my heart and as I was barreling towards 40, not good for my skin.

Then, my father passed away. I ended up staying with my mother for about three months or so afterward to help her take care of things and transition to living without a partner. My mother's house was outside the city limits, out by the lake. No pizza delivery there. Quite by accident, I was eating healthy meals seven days a week. No cheating on the weekends there. Within a month I had lost 10 pounds and by the following month another ten pounds. I realized my "in moderation" attitude had sabotaged my goals.

Are there ways you sabotage your own efforts to better health? Something to ponder.

Some changes are more challenging than others. Keep in mind that your eating habits have been formed throughout your lifetime. Be patient. Have faith in yourself. I feel confident you can do this just like I did.

There are two types of Banned Foods. There are foods you ban for life and then there are foods you ban in certain places or certain times. For example You may ban pie and cake except for holidays only. I did this the first few years and eventually found I didn't even want pie or cake during the holidays. A permanent ban, for life, should be things like carbonated beverages, candy, the bread they bring out before your meal at a restaurant, and the donuts and pastry brought into the office during meetings.

You could do a Banned Foods List for your home. I do not purchase candy, desserts, or sweets, no chips, cookies, snack foods, soda, alcohol, gluten, dairy, nightshades, or soy products to keep at home but when I go to a restaurant I don't worry about the ingredients as much. I still abide by water or unsweetened tea only, no Texas Toast or rolls before or during the meal, and no dessert while dining out.

There are just certain foods that don't belong as a part of a regular diet. Like candy.

Start your Banned Foods List and post it somewhere like the refrigerator or have it on your phone. Add to it as you go along and realize "This is something I shouldn't be eating. It's sabotaging my health goals."

A note to all those with a sweet tooth. You will never get rid of your sweet tooth by replacing real sugar with artificial sugar or even natural sugar. In all my years as a weight loss counselor and a nutritionist, the majority of people who have stopped eating anything sweet tasting for a few months lose their cravings if they intend to stop eating sweets. I grew up eating Hostess cakes and into my mid-thirties continued to eat the pastry and who can say no to a chocolate chip muffin? But, once I went a few months without any sweet-tasting foods, not even fruit, well, that took care of it. I thought I would have pie for Thanksgiving at least but found I had even lost a taste for that. From that day forward even my tea and coffee went unsweetened.

Breakfast Menu

During these 45 days, you will avoid breakfast cereals, hot and cold. No donuts or pastry. No syrup.

Honestly, whatever you choose to eat within an hour or so of rising is considered breakfast so feel free to choose any foods, or combination of foods within this book. But, here are a few obvious suggestions for you.

Against the Grain brand bagel with dairy-free butter or an egg. Limit approved grain-free bagels to just twice a week or less due to the carb count.

Don't forget the Against the Grain Raisin Bagel in the lists above, as well as the Simple Mills Muffin Mixes.

Cauliflower Hash

- ½ cup Fresh cauliflower grated or leftover cauliflower that has been boiled.
- Tablespoon of minced onion
- One egg
- Salt

Whisk the egg and then add the remaining ingredients. Heat a skillet that has been sprayed with nonstick cooking spray (even a nonstick pan), or add just a small amount of oil or dairy-free butter.
Press the cauliflower mixture into the skillet and let brown on one side to a nice golden brown before flipping over, hopefully in one piece. Let the other side brown and enjoy.

Eggs

Eggs any way you like them is always a good choice.

Did You Know?

According to incredibleegg.org on egg nutrition eggs are a great source of protein, riboflavin, Vitamin B12, Vitamin D, Selenium, and Iodine. So very healthy for those with thyroid issues or in need of Vitamin D and B12. Plus, eggs have no carbs and no sugar.

If you are a vegan, or your doctor has you on a no-egg diet please follow your healthcare provider's instructions.

Mushroom Omelet

- 3 eggs
- 1 tablespoons minced onion (optional)
- ¼ of a Portobello mushroom, sliced
- Salt and pepper
- Dairy-free butter

Melt the dairy-free butter in a skillet and add the minced onion. Stirring around until translucent and tender. Remove from skillet. Add sliced mushroom. Fry until tender on both sides and turns a dark brown. Remove from skillet.
Whisk the eggs, adding salt and pepper to taste. Pour into skillet. Use a large enough skillet that the eggs have plenty of room to thin out.

Place a lid on the skillet for 3 minutes over medium heat. Add mushrooms and onion to the entire skillet over the cooked egg. Flip the egg folding one half over the other, like an omelet. Remove from heat, place the lid back onto the skillet, and let rest for 3-5 minutes before serving.

Sweet Potato Hash

Peel and then, using a grater, grate the potato into shreds. Salt and pepper. Spray a skillet with non-stick cooking spray. Press the shredded sweet potatoes into the skillet and allow to brown on the bottom before flipping over. They may not completely stay together. That's okay, just flip so that the browned side is now facing up. Again, press into the skillet and allow to brown. This works best on medium to high heat, usually closer to the medium setting. All stovetops vary.

Variation: Whisk one egg and add to the shredded potatoes, salt, and pepper before adding to the skillet to brown. Be sure the whisked egg and potato are combined well.

Yogurt

About six ounces of plain yogurt.
Yogurt with berries.
Yogurt with nuts and seeds.
Yogurt with nuts and berries!

Flavored yogurts have approximately 26 carbs per serving. Plain yogurt only has approximately 13 carbs per serving.

- Eggs, any style. Scrambled, poached, fried, baked, omelet.
- Simple Mills Bread Mix toast
- Baked Sweet Potato: prepare in the microwave or, wrap in foil and cook overnight in the crockpot.
- Avocado Toast (add a fried or poached egg if you want)
- Nuts, seeds and berries. Top with some Unsweetened Almond Milk and eat with a spoon.
- Simple Mills brand muffin mix.
- Uncured Bacon
- Dairy-free yogurt. Mix the yogurt and the nuts for a complete meal.
- Cauliflower Hash
- Salad

It is quite common for people in Europe to eat a salad for breakfast. Many who visit Paris or Turkey often come back with that very healthy habit.

Think of a salad with hard-boiled eggs and uncured bacon and throw on some fresh avocado. Or, maybe a salad with nuts and seeds and some berries.

Lunch and Supper Menu

Again, like breakfast, lunch is whatever you eat for lunch. If you want to make an omelet then do that. Have leftovers from supper? Sure, just heat and eat. Often I will make an extra piece of fish or chicken when cooking supper just so I know I'll have something readymade for lunch the next day. Extra vegetables are always a great idea for leftovers too.

A reminder to stay away from all grains during this **45 Days To Better Health**. No rice, oats, corn, wheat, or any product made from those ingredients.

A reminder also that even grain-free pasta is a high-carb food and your consumption should be limited.

First, let's talk about vegetables. Vegetables are the healthiest of the food groups. If you are not currently a big fan I hope you will give them another try. Our taste buds change as we become adults and as we age so I encourage you to even try vegetables that you perhaps did not like as a child or in your twenties and give them another chance. Try preparing them differently. I don't like canned spinach but I love fresh and frozen spinach.

Menu Ideas for supper can be anything from the list above or below. Choose a protein if you eat meat or fish and a vegetable. Keep it simple. Do a quick searing, bake, poach, sauté or stir fry. These are all familiar foods and most likely foods you already prepare.

- Steak and baked sweet potato or steak and salad. Steak and roasted vegetables.
- Egg salad, tuna salad, chicken salad
- Vegetables are also one of the most versatile foods.
- Soup
- Stew
- Tacos and burritos
- Roasted chicken, baked chicken, poached chicken, stir-fried chicken

Menu Ideas For Vegetables:

- Soups (broth-based and creamy)
- Stir-fry
- Baked (roasted) in the oven
- In cold salads
- Raw veggies with dip
- In sauces like Alfredo
- Cook them in your crock pot or air fryer
- Slaw made with traditional cabbage or you could use shredded lettuce or shredded broccoli to make slaw. Great as a side dish or on fish tacos.

Vegetables offer you protein, fiber, Vitamin C and more.

You may have noticed the Vegetables list above was missing some popular vegetables. Here is the list of vegetables you should avoid during these 45 days:

- White Potatoes and Red Potatoes (sweet potatoes are okay to eat)
- Eggplant
- Tomatoes
- Peppers (Bell peppers, hot and sweet peppers) Black Pepper is okay.
- By-products of these to avoid like paprika, crushed red pepper

These are nightshades and have been known to cause inflammation in joints as well as aggravate stomach issues for some.

Tobacco is also a nightshade and we encourage you to stop smoking if you have been thinking about it.

Coffee is not a nightshade but is very acidic and can wreak havoc on the stomach. This is one of the reasons I am asking you to abstain from coffee during the 45 days. Even if you are not currently experiencing stomach issues it is still very important to avoid coffee, regular and decaf, during this time.

Beef Stir-fry

- About one pound skirt steak, cut into strips
- Salt and pepper
- ¼ cup Coconut Aminos (Soy Sauce substitute)
- 2 tablespoons lime juice
- 2 tablespoons oil
- 2 garlic cloves, peeled, smashed and minced
- One bunch fresh scallions, chopped
- Six ounces fresh mushrooms, sliced
- Six ounces fresh snow peas

Season the skirt steak with salt and pepper. In a medium bowl combine the Coconut Aminos, lime juice, and garlic. Add skirt steak to the sauce and let marinate for 30 minutes or you could do this the night before or the morning of. Keep in the refrigerator and preferably in a glass container with a lid.

In a large skillet over medium to high heat, heat the oil until hot. Add the beef, shaking off excess marinade. Keep the marinade for later.

Cook the beef until just browned. Skirt Steak beef is generally rather thin and should cook rather quickly.

Remove beef from the skillet and add the marinade. Boil for about five minutes cooking it down. Add mushrooms, scallions, and snow peas. Cook for about two minutes or so. Just until starting to be tender but still stir-fry firm. Return the beef to the skillet with the vegetables and combine.

This is a dish that goes well with a package of frozen riced cauliflower. The sauce seasons the cauliflower nicely.

Cauliflower

Cauliflower Casserole

- 2 cups Mashed cauliflower (best if boiled in chicken broth)
- One pound of Ground beef
- ¼ cup (approximately) chopped onion
- 2 garlic cloves, smashed and minced

Cilantro Lime Cauliflower

- 12 ounces frozen riced cauliflower or fresh cauliflower you have riced or grated.
- 1 tablespoon dairy-free butter
- 1 tablespoon oil
- ½ teaspoon salt
- 4 tablespoons chopped fresh cilantro or parsley
- 2-3 tablespoons lime juice

Melt butter with the oil in a large skillet. Add the cauliflower and stir around until coated well. Add salt. Heat through.

If you want a fluffier light cauliflower remove it from heat now and toss with the lime juice.

Or, you can press it into the skillet and allow it to brown on one side for a crispier cauliflower. Remove from heat, toss with lime juice, and serve.

Cold Riced Cauliflower Salad

Blanch frozen riced cauliflower, drain, and allow to cool and then toss with oil and vinegar. Then you can add your choice of the following:

- frozen peas
- green onions (scallions)

- diced or shredded carrots
- Chopped artichokes (can or jar)
- Olives; your choice

Add a dollop of mayo if you want to add a bit of creaminess. Or you could toss it with oil and lemon juice and add chopped parsley or cilantro.

Mashed Cauliflower

Mashed cauliflower can be quite good. I often get negative reactions to it. Here is my tip to make it tasty to nearly anyone:

Boil a fresh head of cauliflower in chicken broth, not plain water. Drain, mash, and whip like you would potatoes. Add dairy-free butter, garlic, and salt to taste.

Riced Cauliflower

Fresh or frozen works in most recipes. If you want the consistency most like rice choose a fresh head of cauliflower but I find I like the frozen too for the convenience.

Use your riced cauliflower to sauté along with vegetables, ground beef, and chicken. Also, use it for fresh cold salads.

Risotto

A delightful way to use riced cauliflower is to make risotto.

- 2 tablespoons dairy-free butter
- 2 tablespoons oil
- 8 ounces fresh chopped mushrooms
- 1 garlic clove, minced
- 12-ounce riced cauliflower
- ½ cup to ¾ cup chicken broth
- One level tablespoon of arrowroot or cornstarch
- Salt and pepper to taste

Place the butter and oil in a large skillet over medium heat. Add the chopped mushrooms and the garlic. Saute until the mushrooms are tender and starting to turn brown. Go ahead and season with salt and pepper. Leave the pepper out if you prefer.

Add the cornstarch and stir around to coat well.

Add the chicken broth. Stirring constantly. Lower heat just a bit.

Add the riced cauliflower. Continue to stir and add more broth if needed.

Roasted Cauliflower Halves

Remove the stem of a fresh head of cauliflower. Slice horizontally so you have large pieces of cauliflower steaks about ½ inch wide. Brush with oil, salt and pepper. Some people like to add some cumin or garlic powder. Or you can pour some oil on a large flat plate and lay each side of the cauliflower into the oil to coat. Shake off the excess before placing it on the baking sheet.

Place in a pre-heated 425-degree oven. Cook for 15 minutes on one side and 15 minutes on the other for a total time of 30 minutes.

Chicken

If you eat meat, chicken is a healthy, low-carb, high-protein food. It is also versatile. It can be eaten cold or hot. Baked, seared, poached, sautéed, roasted or grilled. You can prepare it on the stovetop, in the oven, in an air fryer, or in a crock pot.

- Chicken soup
- Chicken stir-fry
- Roasted chicken
- Baked Chicken
- Chicken salad

Baked Chicken Breast

- 2 Chicken Boneless chicken breast
- Salt
- Skillet that can go from the stovetop to the oven such as cast iron.
- Non-stick Cooking spray

Spray the cast iron skillet. Salt both sides of each chicken breast while the skillet is getting hot on the stovetop. Sear the fatty topside of the chicken until golden brown which should only take five minutes or less. Turn the chicken over and transfer the skillet to a preheated 375 oven.

Bake 20 minutes for thicker pieces and just 15 minutes for thin cuts. This is only for boneless pieces. Meat with the bone-in would need longer cooking times.

Remove the chicken after set time and allow to rest five full minutes before serving.

Chicken Piccata

- Boneless skinless chicken breasts filleted, sliced horizontally for two thinner pieces if thick. Or, use a mallet and flatten the breast. Salt both sides.

- Arrowroot flour
- Cooking oil
- Chicken broth
- Garlic
- Jar of capers
- Dairy-free butter

Dry your chicken, salt on both sides and lightly coat with the arrowroot.

Heat enough oil to cover the bottom of a skillet and then add chicken pieces.

Brown both sides until a nice golden brown over medium heat. This should only take five minutes or so with thin slices. Remove chicken from skillet

Add about one cup of chicken broth to the skillet and be sure to scrape the bottom of the skillet to loosen any chicken. Add capers and minced garlic. Stir around to heat through. Remove from heat and immediately add the butter and then add the chicken back to the skillet.

You can add lemon zest if you want a lemon flavor and/or chopped scallions are also a nice topping. Serve with a vegetable or grain-free pasta like Banza pasta.

Carb servings, like pasta, should be the smallest portion on the plate.

Chicken Salad

Make it how you normally would, just be sure to use one of the approved mayo's on our list.

Greek Fest Chicken

- 2 Boneless Skinless chicken breast
- ¼ cup black olives (whole or sliced)
- ¼ cup kamala olives (whole or sliced)
- 2 tablespoons chopped onion (optional)
- One can drained and rinsed artichoke hearts
- 1 cup chicken broth
- 2 tablespoons dairy-free butter
- 1 garlic clove, smashed and minced
- 8 ounces fresh mushrooms, sliced (optional)

Preheat oven to 375 degrees.

Salt both sides of the raw chicken. Brown in a hot skillet that has been sprayed with nonstick cooking spray. When both sides are golden brown, transfer out of the skillet to the oven to finish. Bake for 15 minutes.

To the skillet left on the stove, add just a splash of the broth and scrape the bottom to loosen chicken bits if any. Add mushrooms and onions. Stir and allow to cook until just getting tender or changes color. Add garlic, olives, and the artichokes. Your burner should be on medium to high heat but not High. Add the chicken broth and allow to boil and cook down a bit. Add the cooked chicken back into the skillet. Now add the dairy-free butter.

Variation: If you need a bit more substance to the meal you could cook a small amount of pasta. It should be equal to about only half of the

73

number of olives and artichokes. Add cooked pasta right into the dish and stir to coat. You could also choose a small amount of white (Northern) beans. About ½ a can that has been rinsed. My preference is the Northern beans. A really nice dish.

Roasted Chicken

- One whole hen or chicken.
- Salt
- Black pepper (optional)

Preheat the oven to 375 degrees. Remove the neck and gizzard from inside the cavity to discard or, for broth or fried gizzards if you like!

Pat the hen dry with a paper towel. Season well on all sides. You can add other seasonings if you like.

Place on baking sheet breast side up and cover loosely with foil.

Bake in a preheated 375 oven. Allow 15 minutes per pound with foil, plus 20 minutes without foil. Ovens vary so check that your chicken is 165 degrees before eating.

No need for basting. While the hen is baking do not open the door until it is time to remove the foil.

Once you have removed the hen allow to rest at least fifteen full minutes before cutting.

If you are not sure how to cut a chicken there are great how-to videos on the internet.

Smothered Chicken

- 2 raw boneless, skinless chicken breast
- 2 tablespoons dairy-free butter or oil
- 1 heaping tablespoon cornstarch or arrowroot
- 1 bulb fresh garlic, smashed and minced
- 2 cups chicken broth
- Fresh sliced mushrooms (optional)
- Fresh or frozen chopped spinach (optional)

*The mushrooms and spinach are showing as optional because you can use both or just one or the other. Both give you the best dish.

Melt butter or heat oil in a large skillet. Brown chicken on both sides (butterfly for faster cooking). Transfer chicken to a baking sheet to a 375 preheated oven for 15 minutes.

While the chicken is baking, add garlic and mushrooms to the skillet on the stove. Sprinkle the mushrooms in the skillet with cornstarch and stir around to coat. Add half of the chicken broth stirring constantly and add the rest to the consistency you are looking for. Should be the consistency of a sauce or gravy. Add the chicken and spinach and allow all to marry for about five minutes.

Tamarind Baked Chicken

- A pound of chicken pieces or four chicken breasts
- ½ cup parsley or cilantro leaves, finely chopped.
- ¼ cup healthy oil
- ¼ cup Tamarind Paste Concentrate
- ¼ cup chopped scallions
- 1 tablespoon cumin
- One teaspoon salt
- 2 medium garlic cloves, minced or grated

Pat chicken dry and set aside while preparing other ingredients.

Combine the oil, cilantro or parsley, tamarind, cumin, salt, and garlic, in a large bowl. Add the chicken pieces and toss around to coat.

Preheat oven to 350 degrees and let the chicken sit while the oven is preheating.

Arrange the chicken on a baking sheet lined with aluminum foil that has been sprayed with nonstick cooking spray. If you are using bone-in chicken pieces bake uncovered for about 40 minutes and let rest for ten minutes before serving.

If you are baking boneless chicken bake about 20 minutes uncovered and allow the chicken to rest ten minutes before serving.

Serve with an approved vegetable like green beans, asparagus, or a salad.

Condiments Recipes

Chimichurri Sauce (Pesto)

This is a great sauce on tacos or a sandwich while avoiding mayo, mustard, and traditional salsa.

One cup minced flat-leaf parsley or cilantro
2 teaspoons minced garlic
¾ cup oil
Salt to taste

Chop the parsley fine using a knife or use a chopper or food processor. Use a grater or knife to mince the garlic or *buy garlic in a jar that is already minced. Combine the parsley and garlic in a bowl and slowly whisk in the oil. Add salt. This should sit and rest for at least fifteen minutes before eating. Best eaten the same day, room temperature.

*Most of the jarred minced garlic will have citric acid listed as the last ingredient. I find this scant amount is not bothersome. Eat products like this minimally though and choose fresh garlic cloves that you mince yourself whenever possible.

Cucumber Dressing or Dip

- 1 cup mayo
- ½ to whole peeled and sliced cucumber
- ½ teaspoon salt
- ½ teaspoon Dill (fresh or ground)
- One small garlic clove, minced
- Olive oil to dressing consistency (optional)

Place all the ingredients except the oil and garlic into a blender or chopper. Blend just enough to break up the cucumber and blend into mayo. If too thick add oil, a little at a time until the consistency of dressing you like. Fold in the garlic and season again to taste. Place in a glass jar with a lid and refrigerate for at least 30 minutes.

Guacamole

- 2 soft avocados
- Lime juice to taste
- Fresh garlic (optional)
- Salt to taste

Serve with Siete grain-free tortilla chips

Hummus

- Chickpeas (Garbanzo Beans) drained and rinsed
- One large garlic clove, smashed and minced
- 1 tablespoon lemon or lime juice
- ½ teaspoon cumin
- A light shake of sesame oil
- Salt to taste
- Olive Oil

Place beans, lemon juice, cumin, and a bit of salt with the sesame oil in a food processor. Pulse a few times, then add olive oil. Continue to add olive oil until the consistency you want. Fold in the garlic after removed from the food processor.

Serve with raw cauliflower, carrots, and Siete grain-free tortilla chips.

Mayo Dressing

- ¾ cup approved mayo
- 3 tablespoons water or oil
- ¼ teaspoon salt
- A pinch of black pepper (optional)

Combine all of the ingredients. This is a nice opportunity for a jar and lid. Shake well.

Variations: You could optionally add garlic powder, dry dill (my favorite), or even vinegar in place of the water/oil. You could also choose lemon or lime juice in place of the water/oil.

Vinaigrette Salad Dressing

- 1 cup olive oil
- ¼ cup apple cider vinegar or one of your favorites
- ½ teaspoon salt

Mix the three ingredients in a jar, a blender, or in a bowl using a whisk. This is the basic dressing that you could store leftovers in the refrigerator for a week. If you add some optional ingredients like minced garlic do so the day you will serve and allow to marinate for about half an hour. If you find this is too much vinegar add more oil.

If you like a creamy dressing you could whisk in an approved mayonnaise.

I have come to like just oil and salt or for a creamy dressing simply mayo.

Watermelon Salsa

2 cups diced watermelon, about the size of a pea
1 small cucumber peeled and also diced OR minced black olives
½ red onion, diced
Chopped cilantro, parsley or some prefer fresh mint
Juice from one whole lime
Salt to taste

Allow this mixture to marinate together for at least an hour preferably in the refrigerator.

White Pizza Sauce

- 1 cup cashew nuts
- 1 ¼ cup unsweetened almond milk
- 1 tablespoon nutritional yeast
- 1 teaspoon lemon juice
- 1 teaspoon garlic, smashed and minced
- ¼ teaspoon onion powder
- 2 tablespoons oil
- 1 teaspoon salt
- 1 tablespoon basil

First, you will want to prepare the cashews by soaking them in water for at least four hours, or you could soak them overnight. Drain them well then place them in a food processor and pulse several times until the cashews are minced.

Add the rest of the ingredients, except the garlic, to the food processor: the milk, nutritional yeast, lemon juice, onion powder, oil, salt, and basil. Blend until smooth and then fold in the garlic.

This also makes a good pasta sauce. I like to add some frozen chopped spinach when using it as an alfredo for pasta or cooked mixed vegetables. It is especially good on cooked, drained yellow squash.

Ground Beef

Ground beef is one of the most versatile of meats. And, generally more affordable. Add browned ground beef to some broth and vegetables and you have soup! Add it to some sautéed vegetables for a more hearty meal. Don't limit yourself to hot-cooked vegetables either. Add ground beef under or over a bed of lettuce. Think taco salad. I watched a cooking show where they visit restaurants and they share their recipes with the viewers. One Mexican restaurant shared that their taco meat was merely ground beef, onions, and lime juice. I wanted to try this as it doesn't have any nightshades (tomatoes), which I avoid in my regular diet. Now I add cumin for a bit more flavor but it tastes great. This is especially good for those of you told to avoid spicy or acidic foods.

Beefy Green Bean Quick Meal

- ½ pound Ground beef (could easily use one pound if needed)
- One can French green beans, drained
- ½ cup chicken broth
- 4 tablespoons apple cider vinegar
- 2 tablespoons minced white onion
- ½ teaspoon salt

Brown salted ground beef and onion. Add green beans, ½ cup chicken broth, and vinegar. Heat through and serve. A very quick but satisfying low-carb meal.

Ground Beef Patty

Try a ground beef patty steak with a side vegetable or a salad piled on top or underneath.

If you haven't tried the lettuce bun or lettuce wrap I want to encourage you to do so. Find the largest iceberg lettuce and wrap it around your hamburger, turkey burger, or salmon. If others are at the table not sharing in your diet put both traditional buns and lettuce out. You'd be surprised that people want to try it and how much they like it.

Meatloaf

Meatloaf is another friendly food if you can pass on the oats or bread. Just no glutinous binding. If you use fresh ground beef that has never been frozen you can make a meatloaf that will stay together without that binding. Just add seasonings, form, and bake as usual. Instead of a traditional catsup meatloaf go with a brown gravy made with dairy-free butter, cornstarch arrowroot, and beef broth. Add mushrooms or onions to the gravy to top the meatloaf. Instead of bell pepper try scallions.

Quick Beef and Riced Cauliflower

- 1 cup Riced Cauliflower (fresh or frozen)
- 1 pound ground beef
- ¼ cup beef broth
- 1/3 cup Coconut Aminos
- 1 tablespoon apple cider vinegar
- ½ teaspoon ground ginger
- 1 garlic clove, smashed and minced
- 1 teaspoon arrowroot or cornstarch
- Chopped scallions

Place ground beef in a skillet. Salt while still raw. Brown ground beef. As ground beef is almost done, add garlic. Finish browning. Add ground ginger.

In a separate bowl combine Coconut Aminos, broth, and apple cider vinegar.

Sprinkle cornstarch over the ground beef in the skillet. Stir around to coat. Turn the heat up to nearly high and add the liquid from the separate bowl with the broth.

Stir constantly and allow to thicken. As soon as it begins to thicken lower the heat. Add the cooked riced cauliflower. Combine well. Serve with chopped scallions on top.

Taco or Burritos

- One pound ground beef
- ½ teaspoon salt
- 1 teaspoon Cumin
- 2 tablespoons minced onion
- 1 tablespoon lime juice

Season the raw ground beef with salt and cumin. Brown the ground beef and the onion. Add the lime juice last.

For tacos use one of the approved taco shells like the Sieta Brand or Sieta Brand tortillas to make a burrito. Serve with shredded lettuce and Watermelon Salsa you find in the Condiment Recipes.

Pasta

If you have pasta, as we do have a few grain-free pasta on our list, limit your consumption. Even grain-free pasta is a processed food and high in carbs.

If you have pasta, have it at a ratio of just ¼ of your vegetables or protein. Three-fourths of your plate should be vegetables or protein and just one-fourth pasta.

Roast

Whether it is a pork roast or a beef roast, prepare whichever you normally would have. I like to use my crock pot but nowadays we have choices. Leave out the tomatoes and white potatoes, instead choosing, carrots, celery, onions, mushrooms, sweet potatoes, and turnips.

Roasted Vegetables

Roasted vegetables are technically baked vegetables, but they are quite delicious and really easy to make. Toss your sliced, chopped, or whole vegetables with a light amount of oil and salt before spreading them onto a baking sheet. Be sure you do not crowd the vegetables.

Some of the more traditional vegetables to roast are sliced zucchini and yellow squash. Cauliflower florets or cauliflower steaks, mushrooms, whole or sliced, peeled and sliced sweet potatoes, onions, and carrots. Two more that are simply delicious are whole okra (fresh or frozen), and artichokes (canned or jar). Leave the okra and artichokes whole when you bake them. I find frozen okra works just fine.

Salads

There are some prepared salads you can pick up in the produce department. You may have to skip the dressing, tomatoes, and croutons but there are so many to choose from these days. The convenience can't be beat.

Salads are more than just a bed of lettuce with other vegetables tossed in. Think outside the box here and take a look at some of the examples below.

Cucumber salad

Sliced cucumber, thinly sliced radishes, frozen peas. Toss with oil or dressing.

Cucumber Watermelon Salad

- 2 cups cubed watermelon
- 1/2 cup chopped peeled cucumber
- ½ small red onion, thinly sliced
- 2 tablespoons fresh basil leaves
- ¼ cup fresh spinach leaves
- 2 tablespoons olive oil
- 1 teaspoon Red Wine Vinegar
- 1 tablespoon raw organic honey
- A pinch of salt

Combine the vinegar, honey, salt, and garlic in a bowl.
Whisk in the olive oil to combine well.
Toss in the cucumbers, onions, and watermelon until coated.
Fold in the fresh basil and fresh spinach just before serving.

Find foods you can put shredded lettuce on or under.

Get creative with your salads. Add mushrooms, frozen peas, olives, artichoke hearts, sugar snap peas, or pea pods. Add chicken or even ground beef (think taco salad without the taco seasoning. Instead season the ground beef with cumin, salt, and lime juice).

Try fresh spinach leaves with boiled eggs, and chopped scallions.

Lettuce, strawberries and walnuts.

Egg and Avocado Salad

- 2 boiled eggs, peeled and sliced or chopped
- 1 small avocado, peeled and sliced
- Squeeze of fresh lemon juice
- Salt to taste
- 2 tablespoons mayo

Combine all together. This is a great salad for breakfast, lunch, or supper. Add any other ingredient you might like that is on this list. Some like to add a bit of chopped red onion. I like to place the salad on top of chopped or shredded iceberg or romaine lettuce.

Rainbow Salad

Ginger Dressing
- 2 scallions, chopped
- ¼ cup apple cider vinegar
- 1/3 cup approved mayo
- 1 tablespoon fresh ginger root
- ½ teaspoon mustard
- 1/8 teaspoon salt
- Pinch of black pepper (optional)
- 2 tablespoons canola oil

Salad
- 16 ounces thinly sliced or shredded red cabbage
- 8 ounces grated (shredded) carrots
- 1/8 cup parsley or cilantro, chopped

Combine the salad vegetables and then toss with the dressing. Refrigerate for at least an hour before serving. Tossing in cashews or slivered almonds is a nice addition.

Sweet Potato Fries Salad

- Prepared frozen sweet potatoes
- Shredded iceberg lettuce
- Favorite dressing

Prepare the frozen or fresh sweet potato fries. Top with a big pile of shredded lettuce and then top that with your favorite dressing. This is delicious and satisfying.

Tri-Color Chopped Salad

- 2 tablespoons apple cider vinegar
- 3 tablespoons extra virgin olive oil
- Salt and pepper to taste
- 1 cup chopped radicchio
- 1 cup chopped Belgian Endive
- 1 cup chopped Arugula
- ¼ cup nuts (pine nuts, cashews, or pecans work nicely with this dish)

Whisk together vinegar, oil, salt, and pepper. Combine radicchio, endive and arugula in large bowl. Toss with dressing and then add nuts to top.

94

Seafood Menu Ideas

- Baked fish or seafood. Be sure to season before baking and don't overcook.
- Seafood tacos using one of the grain-free taco shells listed above.
- Scallops
- Shrimp. Shrimp is another versatile food. You can sauté it, grill it, bake it.
- Cod and Salmon are excellent choices to season and then bake.

Recipes

Baked Cod with Dill Sauce

- 2 Cod Fillets
- 2 tablespoons oil
- ½ cup approved mayo
- Minced onion
- 2 teaspoons dried dill
- ¼ teaspoon thyme

Preheat the oven to 400 degrees.

In a bowl combine the mayo, dried dill, thyme, and minced onion (optional)

Grease a baking dish and place fish in it covered with the creamy sauce you just made. Lay a piece of foil loosely over the top.

Bake for 10-12 minutes.

Crab Cakes

1 pound fresh lump crabmeat
1 cup of toasted, crumbed, approved bread (ex: Simple Mills)
1/3 cup approved mayo
1 teaspoon chives
½ teaspoon mustard
¼ teaspoon celery salt
½ teaspoon cumin
Juice of one lemon
¼ teaspoon salt

Combine the drained crabmeat, breadcrumbs, mayo, chives, mustard, celery salt, salt, cumin, and juice of one lemon. Combine well, cover, and refrigerate for at least 30 minutes. This allows not only the flavors to marry but the mixture should firm up.

Now you can make the tartar sauce if you want that as a condiment to your crabcakes.

Tartar Sauce

½ cup mayo
Finely chopped dill pickles
About one teaspoon of capers

Mix well, taste. Add a pinch of salt if you wish. Refrigerate until the crabcakes are done.

Preheat the oven to 400 degrees.

Grab the crabmeat mixture and make your patties. About ½ cup each.

Heat oil in a cast iron skillet or oven-safe skillet. Lightly brown the crabcake patties until a nice lightly golden brown on one side before turning. You should see the browning coming up the side of the patty. Cook on just above medium heat. Using a spatula, gently flip the patty and immediately transfer it to the oven, and bake for just 10 minutes.

Garlic Shrimp

One pound peeled and deveined shrimp
2 tablespoons oil
Salt
5 garlic cloves, smashed and minced
3 tablespoons lemon juice
2 tablespoons capers with the brine
2 tablespoons very cold dairy-free butter
½ cup finely chopped flat-leaf parsley
Water

Best to have all of your ingredients out, measured, and ready to go.

Heat the oil in a large skillet over high heat. Once the skillet is hot add the shrimp in a single layer in the skillet. Let cook, without stirring for about one full minute. Season with salt and stir the shrimp. Allow to cook another minute.

Add garlic, lemon juice, capers, and brine, ¼ of the butter, and half the parsley. Stir and cook until the butter has melted and coated all of the shrimp. (just divide the butter into four parts and use one part in this set of instructions)

Reduce heat to low and add the remaining butter. Stir and allow to cook just until the butter has melted. Shrimp should look opaque or translucent.

Remove the shrimp from the skillet leaving everything else. Add a tablespoon of water and stir to combine making sure to scrape the bottom of the skillet.

Add the remaining parsley to serve.

This is a nice, fancy dish that cooks very quickly.

Soup

If you are making soup, gravy, or sauces you can skip the milk and use broth instead for a creamy base.

Creamy Carrot Soup

This will taste similar to tomato soup.

- 2 cups sliced cooked carrots. If you use canned carrots you will want to drain them and rinse them before using. For fresh carrots slice enough raw carrots for two cups and then boil until very tender and then drain. I do not recommend using frozen carrots for this recipe.

- ¾ to 1 cup beef broth
- One tablespoon diced white onion
- One peeled and minced garlic clove
- ¼ teaspoon celery seed
- 1 Tablespoon apple cider vinegar
- Salt to taste

Pour the cooked carrots (cooled) and the broth into a blender and blend until creamy smooth. Pour into a saucepan and add the remaining ingredients. Combine well, cover, and simmer at least 20 minutes. Taste and season to taste if needed.

*Start with the minimum amount of broth so you are sure it will not be too thin. Should be the consistency of tomato soup.

Black Bean Soup

- Black Beans (dry or canned that have been drained and rinsed)
- Chicken broth
- One garlic clove, peeled, smashed and minced
- Tablespoon of minced onion (optional)
- 1 teaspoon Cumin
- 1 teaspoon lime juice
- ¼ teaspoon salt

Place the cooked black beans in twice as much chicken broth. Add the garlic, cumin, onion and salt. Simmer at least 30 minutes. Remove about half of the beans and mash. Return to the soup and combine well. A whisk works well. Add the lime juice. Serve hot.

*Be mindful that this is a high-carb food if you are trying to lose weight and limit your consumption.

I eat about half a serving and pile on shredded lettuce and avocado.

Steak-Ums

Steak-Um and Cabbage Stir-Fry

- Steak-Um thin sliced beef
- 2 tablespoons oil
- 1 cup cabbage, shredded
- ¼ cup sliced onion (optional)
- 1/8 cup beef broth
- 1 clove of garlic, smashed and minced (optional)
- 1 teaspoon salt
- ½ teaspoon black pepper (optional)

Heat oil in a large skillet. Sauté the garlic and beef just until heated through. Add cabbage and onion along with broth, salt and pepper. Bring to a boil and allow the broth to cook down, stirring while cooking cabbage and onion to tender translucent but still somewhat firm.

Variation: Green peas could be added to this dish along with the cabbage. Or you could substitute the cabbage for broccoli and add a dash or two of Coconut Aminos.

Thin Steak and Kraut

- half can sauerkraut
- Equal amount Steak-Um Thin beef slices
- Salt
- Pinch of celery seed

Salt the beef and heat the beef in a large skillet, then add the kraut and celery seed. Combine well and heat through.

Variations: Some people like to add chopped onion.

Vegetables

So many! If you are not a big vegetable eater here is your chance to try and change that. Something we can count on is that with age our taste buds tend to change. So if you didn't like a particular food as a child I encourage you to give it another try. Many people find they like a certain vegetable so long as it is prepared a certain way. Maybe you grew up with canned peas and canned spinach. Yuck! But guess what? Fresh spinach is nothing similar to canned spinach. Even frozen spinach is good compared to canned. I would never eat canned peas but frozen peas are great not just cooked, but especially added to salads, straight from the freezer. Just rinse in water and that will thaw them enough.

Tired of raw carrots and celery? Try sugar snap peas, radishes, and romaine hearts. Don't forget some refreshing cucumber slices too.

Roasted vegetables. If you haven't tried them yet you are missing out on one of the easiest healthiest dishes one can prepare.

If you like Cream of Asparagus soup you can whip it up quickly yourself using approved ingredients. Use cooked asparagus, either fresh or frozen that you have boiled until quite tender, or, you could use a can of rinsed canned asparagus for this recipe. Place cooked (cooled) asparagus into the blender. No need to cook if coming from a can. Add a cup of chicken broth. Blend just enough to break down the asparagus. Transfer to a saucepan. Add seasonings you like, maybe salt and pepper, some garlic, and perhaps a bit of minced onion. Heat through. Always start with the minimum amount of liquid. You can always add more if you prefer it a bit thin.

You could use this same method to make cream of cauliflower or broccoli soup. However, with these two vegetables, I think fresh is best.

Vegetables can also seem like an entirely new dish just by the way they are presented. Try grated carrot slaw or salad. Mix with any other vegetables you like and then toss with approved mayo. I find this works well with cucumber or even grated raw cauliflower.

Do you like water chestnuts? Rinse a can and toss them with grated carrots and rinsed frozen peas. Toss with oil and vinegar, salt and pepper.

Fancy Mash

- Fresh head of cauliflower
- Fresh kale
- Scallions
- 2-4 cups chicken broth
- Large garlic clove, smashed and minced
- Salt and pepper
- Dairy-free butter

Boil cauliflower in chicken broth until quite tender. Also, boil kale until tender. I find it best not to boil them together as they take different amounts of time to cook through. I usually boil the cauliflower, remove it from the broth, then add the kale to that same broth. While the kale is boiling I mash the cauliflower in a food processor. Peel, smash, and mince the garlic and finely chop the scallions.

The amount of kale and scallions will just depend on how large or small your head of cauliflower is. Choose what looks like the right amount to you.

When the kale has cooked until quite tender, drain and then also squeeze out excess water using your hands. Fold the kale, garlic, dairy-free butter, and scallions into the mashed cauliflower. If you would prefer, hold back the scallions and top the dish with them instead. Be sure to taste the mix and season to taste. If you are adding scallions to the top, season first.

Favorite Hot Spinach

My favorite way to prepare cooked spinach:

Toss fresh spinach in a bowl with a minimal amount of healthy oil, salt, and pepper. Spray a large skillet with non-stick cooking spray. Add two tablespoons water and heat it on the stove on high heat. Once the skillet is hot pile all of the spinach into the skillet and immediately place a lid on top. Remove from the heat and allow to sit a full five minutes. Splash a bit of apple cider vinegar on the spinach and toss before serving. This is a nice side dish to any protein. Even an omelet.

Lots of good vegetable articles and recipes on vegnews.com, a plant-based food and lifestyle site.

Roasted Vegetables

Most popular vegetables to toss with oil, spread onto a baking sheet, and bake in the oven:

- Brussels Sprouts
- Onions
- Cauliflower
- Yellow Squash
- Zucchini
- Mushrooms
- Green Beans
- Asparagus

One of my favorite roasted vegetable duos is frozen whole okra and canned artichoke hearts. Rinse the artichoke hearts and place them in a bowl. Toss whole frozen okra in the bowl straight from the freezer. Toss with a small amount of oil and salt until coated. Spread out onto a baking sheet making sure not to crowd. Bake in a preheated 400-degree oven until golden brown.

Spaghetti Squash

I know the most common way to prepare a spaghetti squash is to cut it in half and bake it. I place the whole spaghetti squash in a large pot of water and boil until a paring knife slides easily into the rind. Be sure it is good and tender. Drain. Cut in half and allow to cool. Much easier to cut in half after it has cooked! Using an ice cream scoop remove the seeds from both halves. Then, you can easily remove the rind by turning each half over and just pulling it off. Use a fork to separate the noodles for your dish.

Personally, I like spaghetti squash simply tossed with some dairy-free butter and salt. I will sometimes prepare it one day and have some for breakfast the next morning with a fried egg on top.

Later in the week spaghetti squash with vegetables and perhaps an approved sauce. Especially good sautéed with mushrooms. Added to broth-based soups, tossed with some browned ground beef too!

Re-Introduction of Foods

After you have successfully gone 45 consecutive days limiting your foods to just those above you can begin to reintroduce foods to your diet.

Reintroducing foods should be done methodically. One food group at a time every two weeks.

A reminder of continued good eating habits:

- Continue to choose water as your beverage with your meals.
- Limit coffee consumption and how late into the day you consume it. An example might be no more than 2 cups no later than 10 am.
- Limit or avoid all sugar except for natural sugars from raw honey, agave, and fresh fruit **after** 45 days of restrictive eating.
- Chew food well. Eat slowly.
- Do not overeat. You should try to avoid feeling overly full.
- If you are hungry you should eat something. Choose healthy foods when you do.

I would encourage you to continue to avoid overly processed foods as much as possible. If and when you do eat them write that down and take note of how you feel. Do you notice headaches or bloating? Do you notice being hungry more often? Faux hunger pangs are a common symptom of overly processed foods. So perhaps you try gluten-free pasta but stay away from seasoning packets.

You will want to keep a notebook or at minimum a list of what you reintroduce and when.

This part is very important.

This is how you find out if you can:

- Return To Eating Some or all Foods As A Part Of Your Regular Diet
- Need To Avoid a specific food or food group altogether
- Or, you have a limited tolerance and how often you can enjoy a cheat meal.

Week One and Two Grains

The first week return non-gluten grains. This means oats, rice, and corn, but not wheat. Do this for a full two weeks and assess how you feel. Are you having stomach issues? Are you experiencing bouts of constipation? Are you feeling more fatigued than usual? If any of these answers are yes remove them once again from your diet and see if you feel better.

If you begin having symptoms like constipation, headaches, and stomach issues then stop eating those foods. Note your symptoms in your notebook.

Week Three and Four ~ Dairy

Now reintroduce the avoided dairy foods. Cheese, milk. Once again, note if you have any symptoms. If not continue to eat them. Some dairy can cause bloating, inflammation, nasal congestion, and in some a slowing of the urine stream or difficulty starting the urine stream in the first place. Restrict these foods if you do, otherwise consider these foods okay to consume. Interestingly, some people find they can have cheese and sour cream but not dairy milk. This is when you find out what works best for you. You may not experience any adverse effects from any dairy or you might find you feel best when you avoid dairy altogether.

Week Five and Six ~ Nightshades

Next reintroduce nightshades like tomatoes, potatoes, peppers, and eggplant. Nightshades are likely culprits of joint pain, acid reflux, and for many, headaches.

Week Seven ~ Gluten

Next, let's try gluten. Wheat flour products like pasta, cereal, and bread. I want you to pay special attention to your mental health as much as you do your physical health. Many people report depression, obsessive control thoughts, and uncontrolled anger coming back that they didn't even realize had disappeared when they restricted gluten more than six weeks ago. Gluten might also cause hives or stomach discomfort, brain fog, and morning stiffness among other mental and physical ailments. Also, keep in mind that all gluten products are highly processed and high in carbs.

As far as highly processed foods and sugar, for good health, we should avoid them when possible. Continue to honor your Banned Foods List. I also caution you against soy. Soy wreaks havoc on the thyroid and hormones.

Moving Forward

Here you are. This isn't the end. This is the beginning. I'm excited for you! I'm also proud of you for taking very important steps toward being as healthy as you can. This will serve you well as you age. That counts for those of you in your twenties as much as for those of you in your sixties and beyond and every age in between.

I hope you have learned something positive about yourself over these last couple of months. That you really can be self-disciplined. It's easier than you thought to make healthy food choices and perhaps you found you like vegetables? I hope so.

I want to encourage you to choose a healthy food every time and if a cheat meal sneaks itself in don't worry about it. Let it go. Remember that so long as healthy foods rule the majority of your regular day-to-day diet you will be fine.

I hope you have cut down on your sugar intake. If you are still having some issues with that please stick to it! Remember that the best way to get rid of a sweet tooth is to go for a period of time without eating anything that tastes sweet.

Most people find it very helpful to know that they don't have to read long ingredient labels or understand what all those long words mean. If you see a long ingredient label just put it back. Those foods are never healthy and are always overly processed.

I also want to encourage you to keep that Banned Foods List! This can be one of the most helpful tools you have.

Exercise and sleep also play a crucial role in a healthy lifestyle. These last few months hopefully found you sleeping better and with more energy, less fatigue just an overall better feeling of wellness. Many find they feel better mentally. Did you find that?

Most importantly I hope you realize that you have more control over your health, physical health, and mental health than you realized.

ABOUT THE AUTHOR

amazon.com/author/paulachenderson